S15470   612.3   Ward, Brian R.
612.3 Ward, Brian R.
WAR   Diet and nutrition
        Diet and nutrition

   $10.90
        $10.90

DATE			

DIET
AND NUTRITION

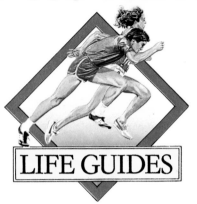

LIFE GUIDES

DIET AND NUTRITION

Brian R. Ward

Series consultant:
Dr Alan Maryon-Davis
MB, BChir, MSc, MRCP, FFCM

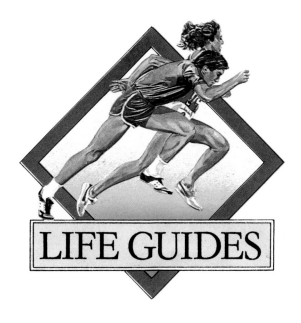

LIFE GUIDES

Franklin Watts
London · New York · Toronto · Sydney

First published in Great Britain in 1987 by
Franklin Watts
12a Golden Square
London W1

First published in the USA by
Franklin Watts Inc.
387 Park Avenue South
New York, N.Y. 10016

First published in Australia by
Franklin Watts Australia
14 Mars Road
Lane Cove
New South Wales 2066

UK ISBN: 0 86313 452 1
US ISBN: 0-531-10259-9
Library of Congress Catalog Card No: 86-50357

Design: Howard Dyke

Picture research: Anne-Marie Ehrlich

Illustrations: Dick Bonson, Penny Dann, Howard Dyke

Photographs:
Chris Fairclough 20, 31
Howard Dyke 22, 24, 35
Sally and Richard Greenhill 7
Hutchison Library 11, 27
Mike Newton 12-13, 15, 16-17, 21, 26, 33, 36, 37, 39
Zefa 19, 28

Home economist: Ellen Nall

Printed in Belgium

Contents

Introduction

Why do we eat? And why do we eat *what* we eat? We need food to build the **cells** and tissues which make up our bodies. This food must contain the right substances or **nutrients** to ensure that our bodies grow properly and are maintained in good health. But there are very many ways of eating these essential nutrients, and people throughout the world have their own ideas about what makes an appetizing meal. We can obtain the proper mix of nutrients in many different ways, by eating a wide variety of foods. All contain the building blocks of life, though in varying proportions.

For this reason, it is important to us that food is appetizing. The appearance, taste, smell and familiarity of food are all important to our enjoyment of a meal. Most of us become used to a particular type of food when we are children, and only begin to experiment with different foods as we get older.

Unfortunately not all of our food is necessarily "good" for us, especially if we come to rely too much on fast foods or "junk" foods.

Eating provides us with all the nutrients we need, but it is also an important social part of our lives. Mealtimes are when young children can learn to try new and unfamiliar foods that improve the range of their diets.

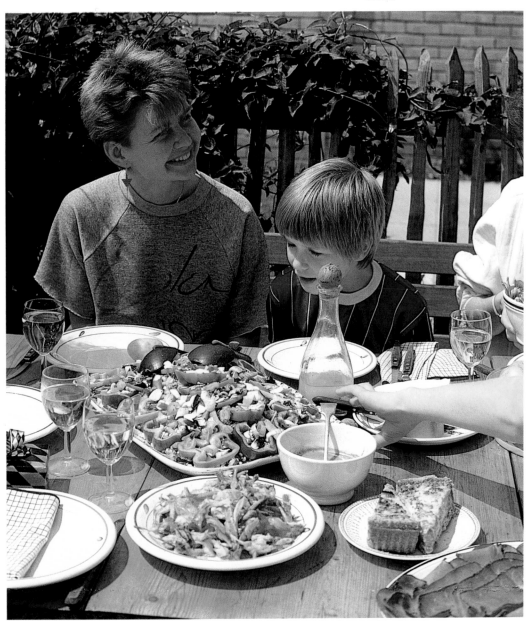

Eating for health

Our diets consist of a mixture of meat, fish, dairy products, vegetables and cereals. These foods contain **protein**, **fat**, **carbohydrates**, **fiber** and **minerals** in different proportions.

Protein is the chief building material of the body and our muscles are largely made up of it. It can be used to provide energy.

Fat is also an energy source. Its other important function is to act as insulation, which is why we have a layer of fat beneath the skin.

Carbohydrates provide the main energy source for the body. They are made up of different kinds of **starches** and **sugars**, and are found in such foods as bread, potatoes and cereals. Sugar itself has no nutritional value, although it is a source of energy.

Fiber is also a type of carbohydrate, made up of the indigestible parts of plant foods. It passes through the digestive system unchanged, but helps to make the solid waste, or **feces**, bulkier and easier to pass.

Minerals are needed in small quantities and are important for growth and the building of bones and teeth.

This meal provides a
reasonably well balanced
mixture of foods. It contains
meat and fresh vegetables,
but rather too much fat and
sugar.

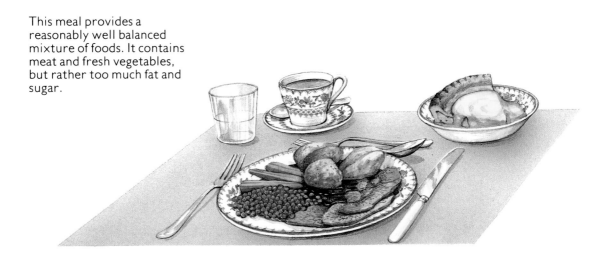

The type of meal produced
by "fast food" restaurants
usually contains large
amounts of fat, salt and sugar
— all of which should be
reduced in a healthy diet.

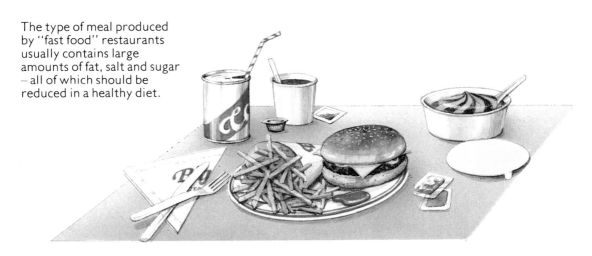

This Chinese meal contains
very little animal fat. It is
rich in fiber, and low in
sugar.

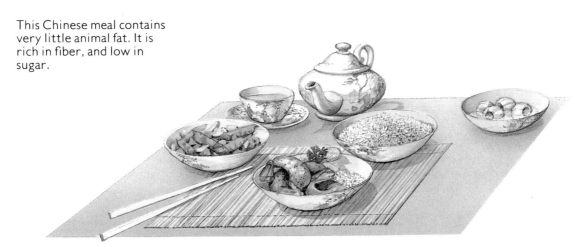

Food and ill health

We cannot live without food, but eating the wrong foods, too much food, or too little food can all contribute to poor health.

In the developed countries many health problems are due to eating too much of the wrong types of food. Sugar, for example, is known to be the cause of **dental decay**. In countries where sugar consumption is low, dental decay is rare.

Diseases of the heart, **strokes** and high blood pressure are all associated with a poor diet. Eating too much fatty food can cause the **arteries** to become clogged, leading to serious illness such as a heart attack. Poor diet is even more damaging if there is a family history of diseases of the circulation, and even worse if a person smokes.

Overeating or eating the wrong types of food can cause weight problems or **obesity**. This is a serious concern in the Western world, where very many people, especially children, are overweight. This can put a strain on the heart and can aggravate diseases such as **diabetes** and **arthritis**.

Opposite

Most of us are lucky enough to be able to select the kind of food we like to eat. But for many people in poorer parts of the world, any type of food is welcome. Apart from the effects of starvation, malnutrition causes many other forms of ill health.

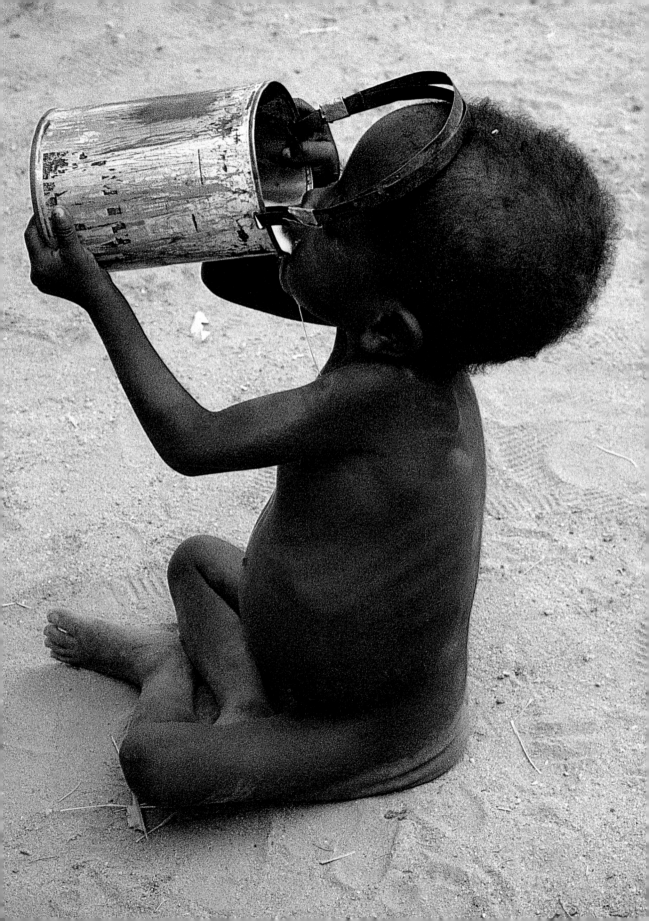

Protein – building the body

Proteins are complicated substances
which make up much of the body tissues.
Living cells are mostly composed of
protein, and many of the substances
produced in the body are also proteins.
Yet protein cannot enter the body
directly from the food we eat. Instead, it
is broken down during **digestion** into
simpler substances called **amino acids**.

All the sources of animal
protein shown here also
contain fat. Protein from
plant sources, like cereals,
nuts and **legumes** – beans,
lentils and peas – contains a
less harmful type of fat, and
they provide a much cheaper
source of protein than meat.

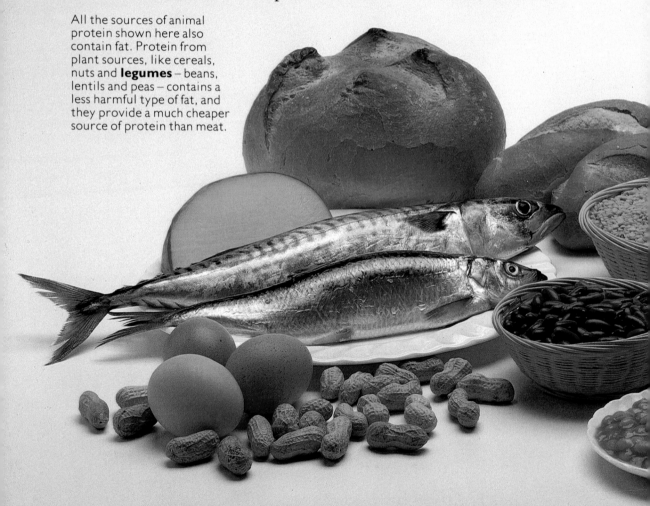

We must obtain these essential amino acids from the food we eat, as our bodies cannot manufacture them. Poultry and fish are good sources of protein, but other animal products like milk, butter, cheese and eggs are also rich in protein.

Animals are not the only source of protein. Plant protein is just as nutritious and usually contains less of the harmful types of fat.

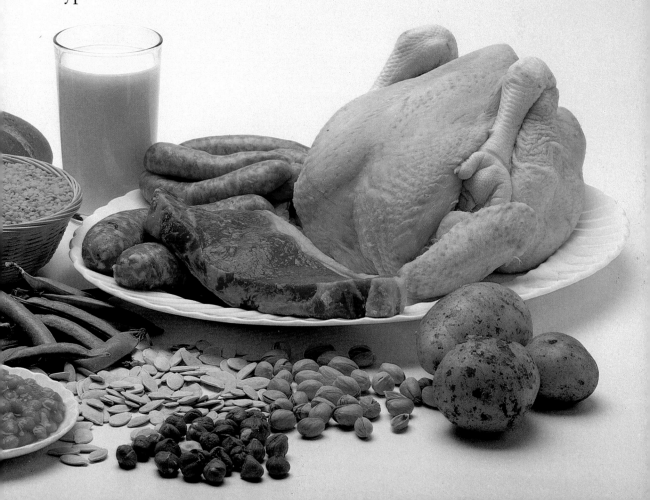

Fats and oils

Fat is a very important energy store for the body. It can be broken down to provide energy and keep the body running if food is in short supply. Fortunately, we seldom need this emergency energy store, but if our body fat builds up to unnecessary levels, it causes overweight or obesity.

Fatty substances in the blood can gradually become deposited on the walls of blood vessels, narrowing them and interfering with blood flow. For this reason, heart attacks and other diseases

All of the diseases shown in this diagram have been associated with eating foods containing too much saturated fat. It is thought that these diseases can be avoided by cutting down on fat intake in the diet.

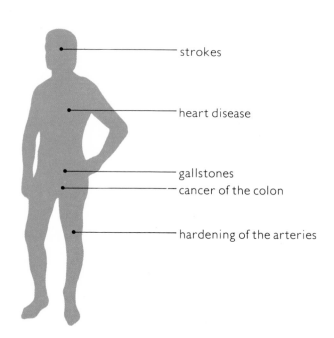

strokes

heart disease

gallstones
cancer of the colon

hardening of the arteries

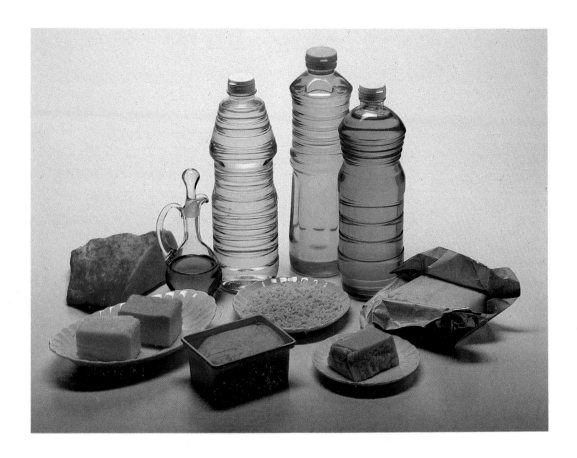

of the circulation are more common in people who eat large amounts of fat. In places like Japan and Africa, where little fat is eaten, heart disease is uncommon.

Fats can be of several types (oils are simply liquid fats). Doctors believe that the risks from a high-fat diet are due mainly to a type of fat called **saturated** fat. This is the fat found mainly in meat and dairy produce, though it is also found in some vegetable fats. Most vegetable fats and oils are **polyunsaturated**. This type of fat does less damage to the arteries and heart.

All of these fats and oils are commonly added to the food we eat or used in cooking. Animal fats, such as butter and lard, are saturated fats, but most vegetable oils, such as corn oil and soybean oil, are polyunsaturated.

Coping with fat

At present, we get nearly 40 per cent of our energy supply from fat. Fat has a high energy content and if we do not burn it all up, we are likely to put on weight.

Doctors believe that this high-fat diet, particularly saturated fat from meat and dairy products, increases the risk of heart disease. Many doctors recommend that our fat intake should be reduced – on average by about a quarter.

All meat contains saturated fat, even if

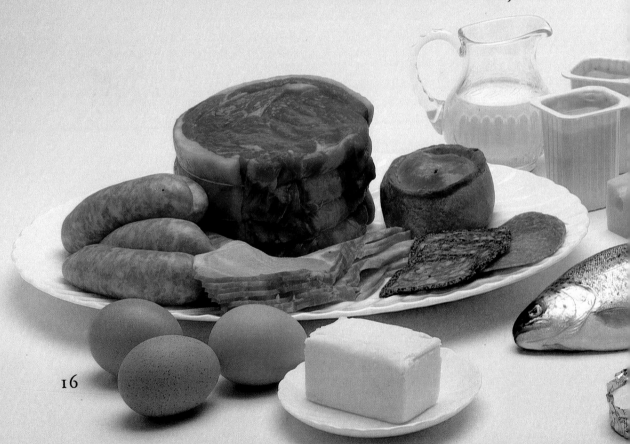

it appears to be lean. This "hidden" fat is also present in many foods like potato chips. Fat is used in most types of cooking, but it is quite easy to substitute the safer polyunsaturated types such as soybean, corn or sunflower oil.

When possible, eat broiled food rather than fried, and trim off any obvious fat from meat.

All of these foods contain significant amounts of fat. The fat content is obvious in foods such as meat, but pastry, cookies and desserts also contain large amounts of fat. Avocados also have a high fat content – this is very unusual for a fruit.

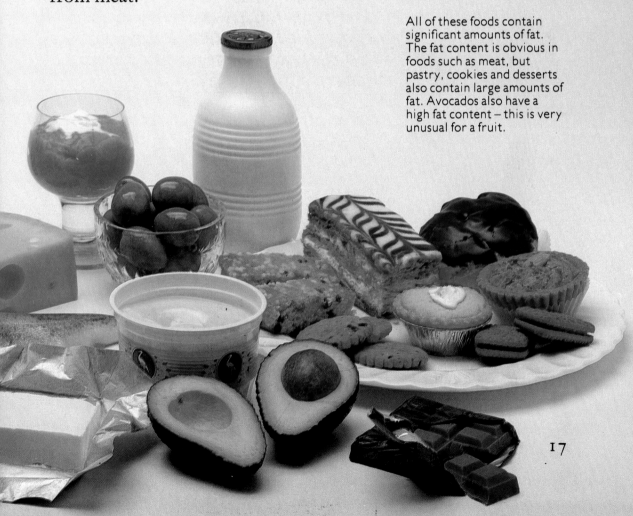

The sweet tooth

Sugar is added in large amounts to many prepared foods. Smaller quantities are naturally present in fruit. Unfortunately the highest levels of sugar are found in the snacks and treats most enjoyed by children, who are especially at risk from tooth decay caused by sugar.

The only practical use for sugar in the body is to provide energy. But starchy foods (like bread, potatoes and rice), fat and protein can provide the energy we need. The reason we use sugar is for its pleasant flavor. At least half of the sugar we consume is in prepared foods or drinks; the balance is what we sprinkle on our food.

Too much sugar, like fat, is a major cause of weight problems. Eating or drinking sugary things too often is also the cause of tooth decay.

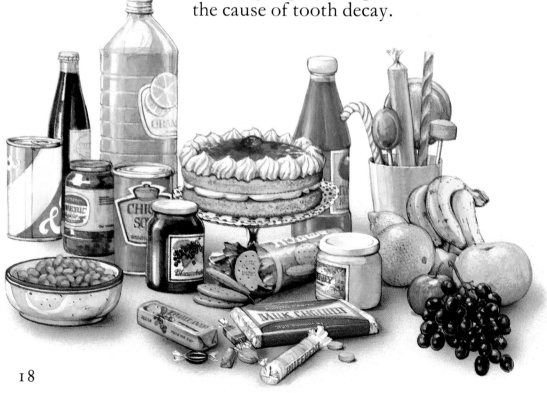

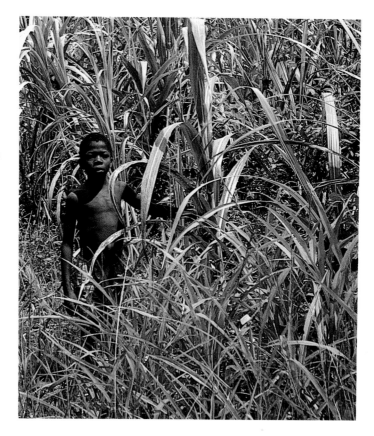

Sugar is an important crop in many parts of the world. Sugar cane (left) is grown in warm, moist climates, while sugar beet is grown as a root crop in cooler areas.

So just as with fats, health authorities have recommended that we cut down on sugar; on average reducing it by at least half.

How can this best be done? The taste for sugar is a mild addiction, but it is one which can be quite easily broken. People who have given up taking sugar in coffee or tea usually come to dislike the sweet taste within a few weeks.

You should also try to cut down on the "hidden" sugar in candy bars and soft drinks. If you get hungry between meals, try nuts, raw vegetables such as carrots, or fresh fruit instead.

Eating too much sugar can result in obesity, which can itself lead to other health problems such as high blood pressure and diabetes.

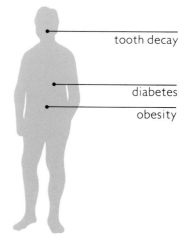

tooth decay

diabetes

obesity

The fiber factor

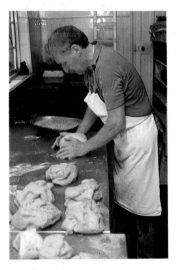

Bread is a staple part of our diet. Changing attitudes to healthy eating are persuading bakers to switch back to wholewheat bread. Make sure it is true wholewheat and not just white bread with added bran and coloring.

Opposite

Fresh fruit, vegetables, nuts and cereals all contain large amounts of fiber. Wholewheat bread contains three times as much fiber as white bread because the flour has not been refined. Similarly, brown rice and wholewheat pasta have higher fiber levels than the refined varieties.

Sugars are members of a group of chemicals called carbohydrates. Sugars are called simple carbohydrates because they can be absorbed directly into the body. Complex carbohydrates, like starches, cannot be absorbed in this way. They are turned into sugars during digestion and are then absorbed.

Other carbohydrates are completely indigestible, and these make up an important part of our diet known as fiber. Fiber consists of the indigestible cell walls of vegetable foods. It passes right through the digestive system unchanged, but it helps to make the solid waste, or feces, soft and bulky.

Fiber is found in many foods that have not been processed or refined. Wholewheat bread, for example, contains all the original fiber from the grain. Breakfast cereals are another useful source of fiber, but you should check to make sure that you have a high-fiber variety. Fruit and vegetables are rich in fiber, although the amounts and types of fiber may vary.

Meat contains *no* fiber at all, which is why a balanced meal needs to contain vegetables as well as meat.

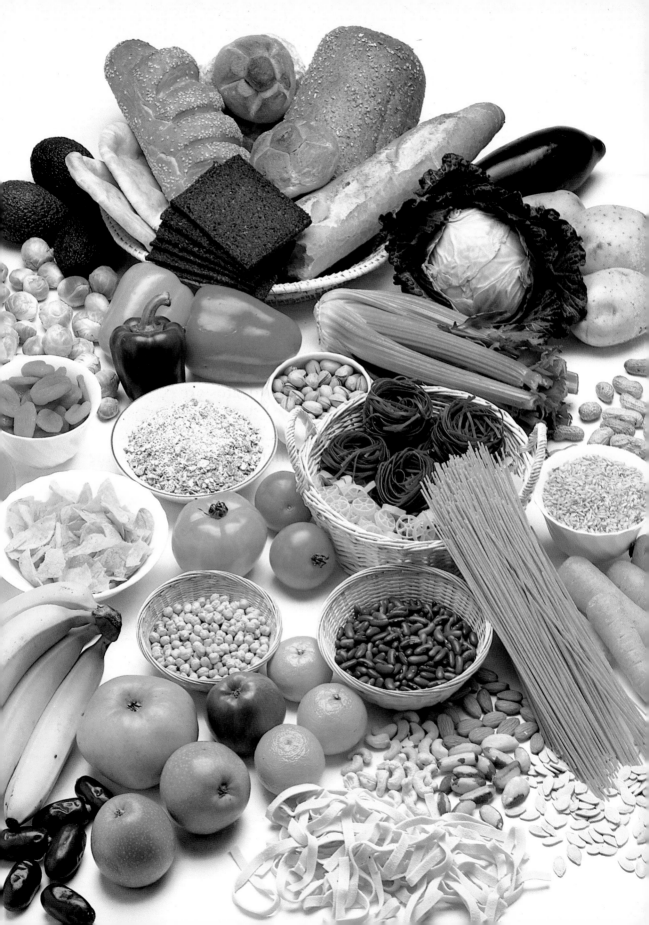

Health and fiber

Most health recommendations are to cut down on foods we normally eat, but doctors and dietitians are advising us to increase our fiber intake.

Food processing and refining remove the fiber from much of the food we eat. This lack of fiber in our diet is responsible for various diseases and considerable ill-health.

Being indigestible, fiber fills out the intestine, and makes the feces easier to pass. Without adequate fiber, the feces become hard, and **constipation** develops. This in turn can lead to other

There is now no difficulty in buying ordinary foods containing plenty of fiber. High-fiber foods are sold in all supermarkets, as well as in the growing number of health food shops. However, it is better to eat food naturally rich in fiber than to add extra fiber to an unhealthy diet.

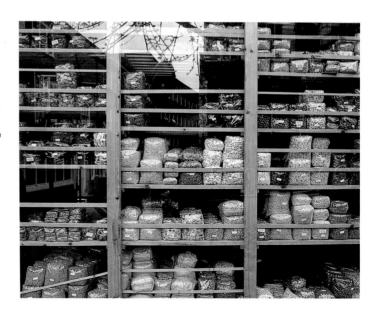

disorders of the **bowel**, such as **diverticulitis** and **hemorrhoids**. Lack of adequate fiber has also been implicated in serious diseases like diabetes and bowel cancer.

A further benefit of fiber is that by filling up the stomach, we feel less hungry, and tend not to overeat. A high-fiber diet, though it looks bulky, will contain relatively few **Calories**, so it is a useful aid to weight control.

Quite recently it has been realized that fiber or roughage in our food plays an important role in keeping us healthy. Several diseases, some very serious, have been associated with eating diets that contain insufficient fiber.

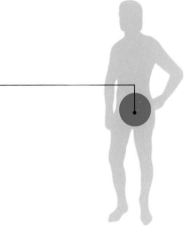

Lack of fiber causes constipation and can sometimes lead to a disease called diverticulitis.

I Waste in the bowel is squeezed along by contractions in the wall of the bowel.

2 If the diet contains little fiber, the waste is less bulky. It becomes hard, and the bowel must work harder to push the waste along.

3 If the bowel has to squeeze too strongly, its lining may burst out into little pouches called diverticula, which can become painfully inflamed.

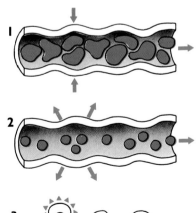

Vitamins – who needs them?

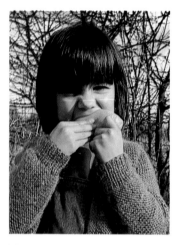

Many of the vitamins we need are found in fresh fruit. Some vitamins are destroyed during cooking, so it is important that you do not rely too much on precooked convenience foods. If you can eat plenty of fresh fruit and vegetables, you will not need vitamin tablets.

Vitamins play an essential part in the body chemistry, helping in many important chemical reactions.

Vitamins are obtained from a wide variety of foods. The body needs only very tiny amounts of vitamins, and a balanced diet will include all of these.

Some vitamins dissolve in the water within the body, and so can be lost in the **urine**. For this reason we need fairly large amounts of the water-soluble vitamins B and C to replace the losses. Other vitamins, like A and D, dissolve only in fat, and so can be stored for long periods in the liver. They are only needed in minute amounts.

Many people believe that they should take extra vitamins, and this has led to a huge vitamin industry, producing millions of vitamin tablets each day. But do we need these extra vitamins?

There is absolutely no evidence that taking vitamin supplements is "good" for you, provided, of course, you are eating a sensibly balanced diet. Vitamin supplements may be needed by the elderly, or during pregnancy, or sometimes after an illness, but the doctor will advise if they are necessary.

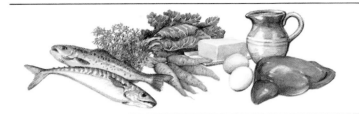

Vitamin A
Found in oily fish, vegetables (especially carrots and spinach), liver and dairy products. Needed for healthy growth, and to keep skin and eyes healthy.

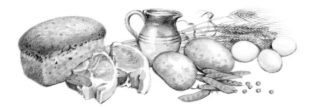

B vitamins
Found mainly in cereals, leafy vegetables, liver, eggs and milk. Needed to help release energy from our food, for healthy growth, and to keep skin healthy.

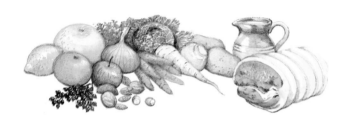

Vitamin C
Found in fruit and vegetables, especially if fresh. It helps to maintain the proper connections between cells. Because it cannot be stored in the body, we need vitamin C every day.

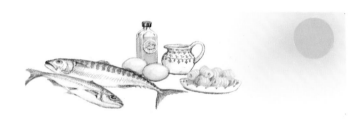

Vitamin D
Found mostly in oily fish, eggs and dairy produce, and made in small amounts by the effects of sun on the skin. Controls the amounts of mineral available for bone formation, which is important in childhood.

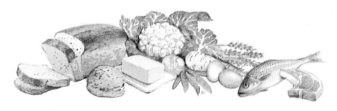

Vitamin E
Found in many foods, especially whole cereals and green leafy vegetables. Needed for cell growth and wound healing.

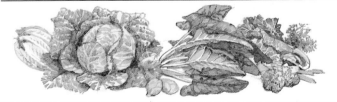

Vitamin K
Found in green vegetables, Vitamin K is very important in helping blood clotting, which stops the loss of blood from wounds.

Down with salt

The body uses many minerals. **Calcium**, for example, is found in milk, and it is very important in growing children as bones develop. Another mineral, **iron**, is used to make the red pigment in blood.

The most common mineral in the body is **sodium chloride**, or salt. Salt is essential for health, but there are risks from taking too much salt, which can lead to dangerously high blood pressure levels. On average we take in ten times as much salt as we need, and health experts

Salt is a common food additive, used for its own flavor, and to enhance the taste of other foods. It is also added to prepared foods as a preservative. We can taste salt in foods like potato chips, but it is added in varying amounts to some unexpected foods. All the foods shown in this picture contain quite large amounts of salt.

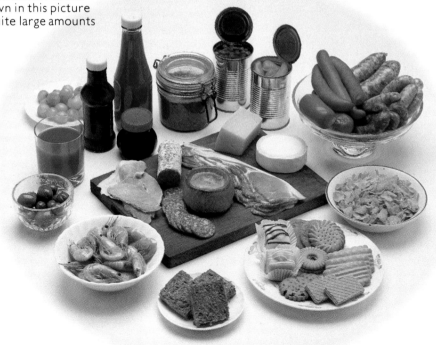

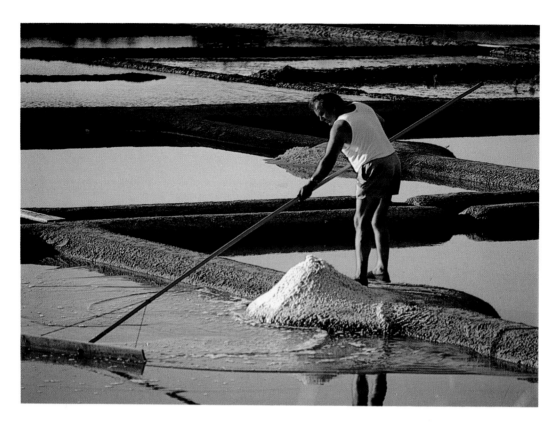

have recommended that we cut our salt intake by half.

Like sugar, we take salt because the flavor is pleasant. Salt actually improves the taste of some foods, and it is added in large amounts to most cooked foods. Salt is present in bread and even in sweet foods such as cookies, as well as being naturally present in meat and fish.

Like sugar, adding salt to food is a habit. It is sensible to taste food before sprinkling on extra salt – it may not be needed. Try to avoid or cut down on salty snacks, and look in the listings on pages 43–5 to find the salt levels in your favorite foods.

Our salt-rich diet is thought to be partly responsible for strokes and heart disease caused by high blood pressure. Doctors regard these as largely preventable if we improve our diet.

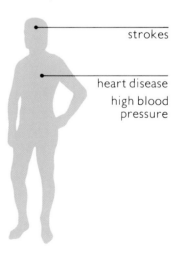

strokes

heart disease
high blood
pressure

Energy and obesity

Starches, sugar and fat are the main sources of energy for the body, although proteins can also be used as fuel. These substances are broken down chemically to release energy, which is then used to power the muscles and all other body systems.

The amount of energy we actually need varies widely. In childhood and adolescence our energy needs are very high, because our bodies are growing.

Sumo wrestlers in Japan deliberately build up their body weight by eating enormous amounts. Because they exercise a great deal, some of this extra weight is muscle.

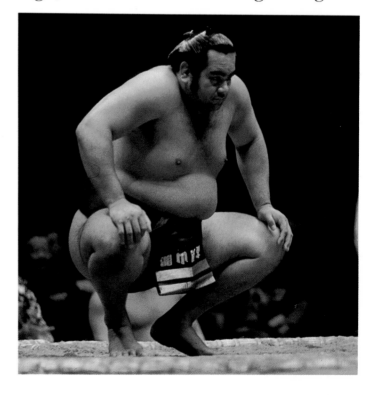

While you are sleeping, your body uses only enough energy to keep the body systems functioning gently. You will use about 65 Calories per hour while you sleep.

At a busy desk job, or while driving or cooking, the body burns 100 Calories each hour.

While jogging or playing football, the body uses 400 Calories per hour, but in a competitive sport such as running, squash, or swimming, Calorie consumption goes up to 650 Calories per hour.

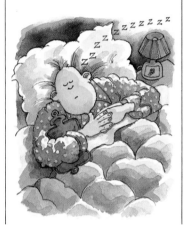

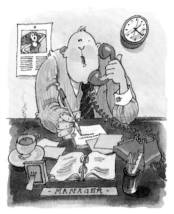

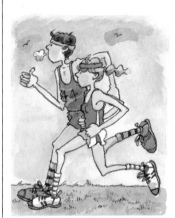

Men tend to use more energy than women, and active people also have high energy demands.

If we do not use all the energy provided by our food, the excess is stored away in the form of fat. Regular exercise burns off some of the excess fat, but most people are unable or unwilling to exercise enough to lose much weight.

Different foods can produce different amounts of energy, and those containing large amounts of sugar or fat are the most energy-rich of all. Their energy content is measured in Calories, and calculation of the energy content of meals is the basis for most weight-reduction diets.

A healthier diet

This is a comparison between our present diet (*top*) and that recommended for improved health (*bottom*). Both diets supply the same amount of Calories, but the balance of nutrients they contain is different.

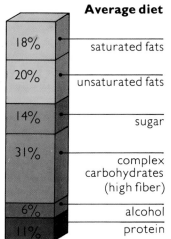

Average diet

18%	saturated fats
20%	unsaturated fats
14%	sugar
31%	complex carbohydrates (high fiber)
6%	alcohol
11%	protein

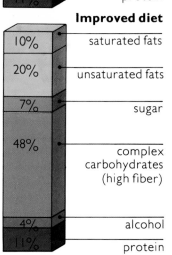

Improved diet

10%	saturated fats
20%	unsaturated fats
7%	sugar
48%	complex carbohydrates (high fiber)
4%	alcohol
11%	protein

The World Health Organization and several other medical authorities have recently made recommendations on ways to make our diet much more healthy. These suggestions include:

Fat: cut down total by 25 per cent, and cut saturated fats by half.

Sugar: cut down by 50 per cent.

Salt: cut down by up to half.

Fiber: increase by 50 per cent.

What do these changes mean? In the short term, it means less tooth decay and obesity, and in the long term, it should enable people to live longer, healthier lives.

Healthier eating means making some small changes in your eating habits. You don't need to sprinkle extra salt or sugar on food, or take sugar in coffee or tea. Switching to fruit instead of eating candy and cookies will increase your fiber intake and decrease sugar and salt.

Not surprisingly, some parts of the food industry do not want any changes in our diet. But as doctors find out more about the effects of eating the wrong foods, it becomes clear that we should cut down on certain foods and switch to healthier alternatives.

Healthy eating should be part of education. Young children often prefer the fried and salty foods traditionally supplied by schools at lunch time, and need educating to eat a much healthier and better balanced diet.

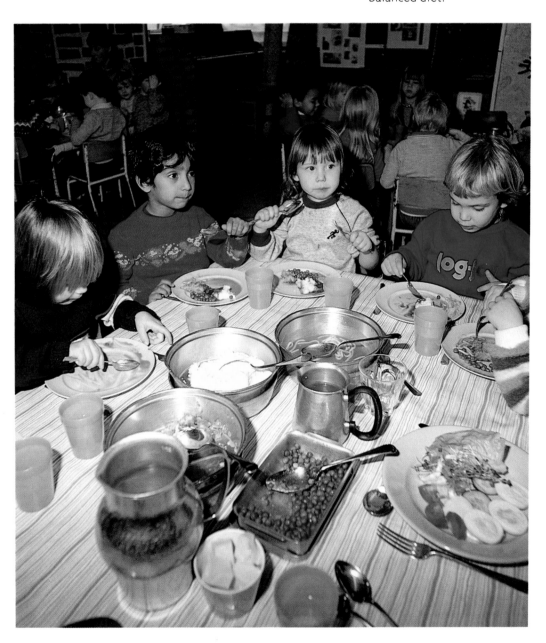

Alternative eating

It is quite easy to adjust your eating habits to make your diet healthier, but some people choose to make more extensive changes to their way of eating.

Vegetarianism is growing in popularity, and most vegetarian diets can form the basis of healthy eating. Vegetarian diets can vary in several ways. In the simplest form, vegetarians avoid only red meat. Others exclude poultry, and some also avoid fish. More rigorous vegetarians refuse all dairy products such as milk, butter and cheese, as well as eggs. They will eat only food that comes from plants.

Some people adopt these diets because the thought of eating animals disturbs them. Others become vegetarian for health reasons, or for religious reasons. But whatever the reason, a vegetarian diet tends to be richer in fiber and lower in saturated fats, and is therefore healthier than our traditional diet. Vegetarians can obtain all the nutrients they need from cereals, legumes, nuts, fruit and vegetables. Such a diet may need careful adjustment to make sure that it contains the proper amounts of protein.

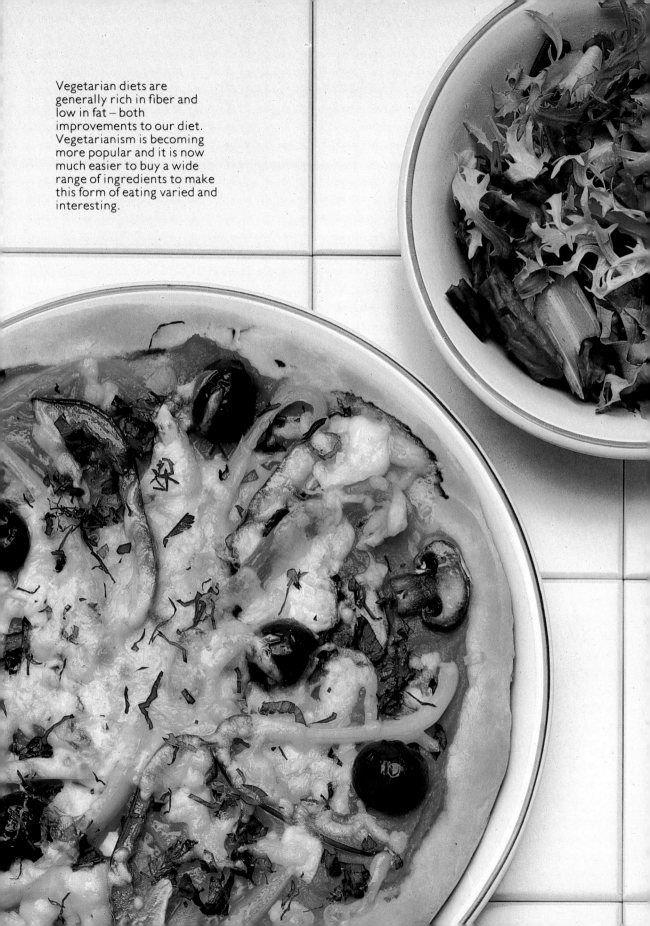

Vegetarian diets are generally rich in fiber and low in fat — both improvements to our diet. Vegetarianism is becoming more popular and it is now much easier to buy a wide range of ingredients to make this form of eating varied and interesting.

Ethnic eating

We are becoming much more international in our taste in food. The interest in food from different countries is partly due to immigrant populations who have established their own restaurants and food stores, but foreign travel also introduces people to new ways of cooking. Spaghetti, frankfurters and chili were once "foreign" foods to many of us, but they are now considered to be everyday foods.

Often these imported foods are healthier than our traditional ones, at least when they are eaten in moderation, and they provide variety and a change in diet. Chinese food, for example, is often fried, but only very lightly in tiny amounts of oil, so it is low in fat and usually contains large proportions of high-fiber vegetables. The olive oil used in Italian cooking is unsaturated, so it is less dangerous to the heart. Pasta, too, provides fiber, especially if it is the wholewheat variety.

Most foods coming from sources other than North America or Europe tend to contain unrefined flour or cereal. Often they are high in fiber and low in animal fat.

Opposite

Foods from many different parts of the world can be found in foreign or specialized food stores, and they can provide interest and variety in our diets.

34

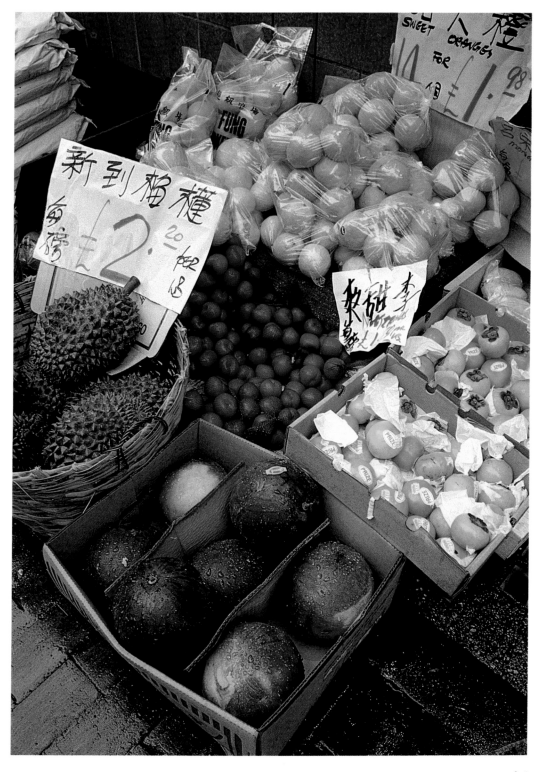

Processed or natural?

This ordinary convenience meal is typical of what is thought to be wrong with our existing diet. It is very low in fiber, and contains large amounts of fat, sugar and salt, as well as a large range of artificial colorings, preservatives and other additives.

Is there such a thing as a "health food"? There is no known food which has a tonic effect, despite the claims of some of the suppliers. There are foods which contain more or less of certain nutrients, but it is the balance of all the food you eat which makes your diet healthy or unhealthy. What does vary is the level of vitamins in foods which have been processed in some way, as some vitamins are destroyed by prolonged cooking. Foods which have been deep frozen for a long time may change in taste or appearance, though there is usually no change in the nutritional value.

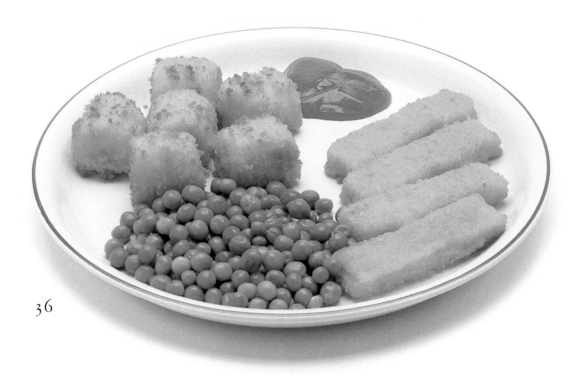

Food is processed for many reasons. Processing may preserve food, allowing it to be eaten out of season. It can do away with the need to clean and prepare the raw ingredients. Processing can also disguise scraps of food which are otherwise unusable. Shreds of meat left on the bone, for example, are often processed to make pies or sausages. Meat substitutes such as soybean are sometimes included in the process.

But for most people, processed food is simply for convenience. If they have time to prepare them, most people prefer fresh meat and vegetables.

A meal prepared from fresh ingredients usually has a much better balance of nutrients. This meal contains plenty of fiber, and the lightly cooked vegetables have retained their vitamins. Only a little salt has to be added to the water in which they are cooked and there is no added sugar. The broiled fish provides protein that is low in fat.

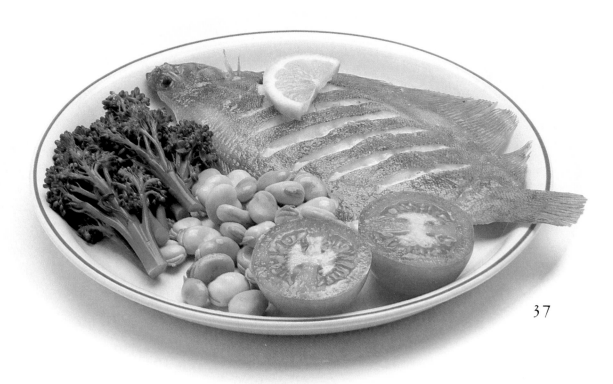

Read the label!

There are strict regulations controlling what can be put into processed foods, including candies and beverages. The ingredients must be listed on the label, but the list itself can be deceptive.

"Vegetable oil," for example, may be a relatively harmless polyunsaturated oil, but it is much more likely to be cheaper saturated oil. Unless it is specifically labeled as "high in polyunsaturates," margarine may be largely saturated animal fat.

The list of ingredients will tell you whether a processed food contains added sugar or salt, but not how much. The label should also list the colorings, preservatives and other substances that have been added. All of these have been tested and approved, but in each country the authorities have come to different conclusions about what is safe.

Why are these **additives** used? Preservatives are obviously useful, but colorings are often unnecessary. The manufacturers give the consumer what they believe the consumer wants. If you *don't* want these additives, avoid buying foods containing them.

Opposite

This Black Forest cake is not quite the attractive dessert it appears. The sponge cake, its filling and the decorative trimmings each contain a large amount of additives – 23 in all! The additives include colorings, emulsifiers (to keep fat well mixed in the synthetic cream), stabilizers, preservatives, starches and citric acid. This is why it's always best to read the label – but the law does not always insist that every ingredient is listed.

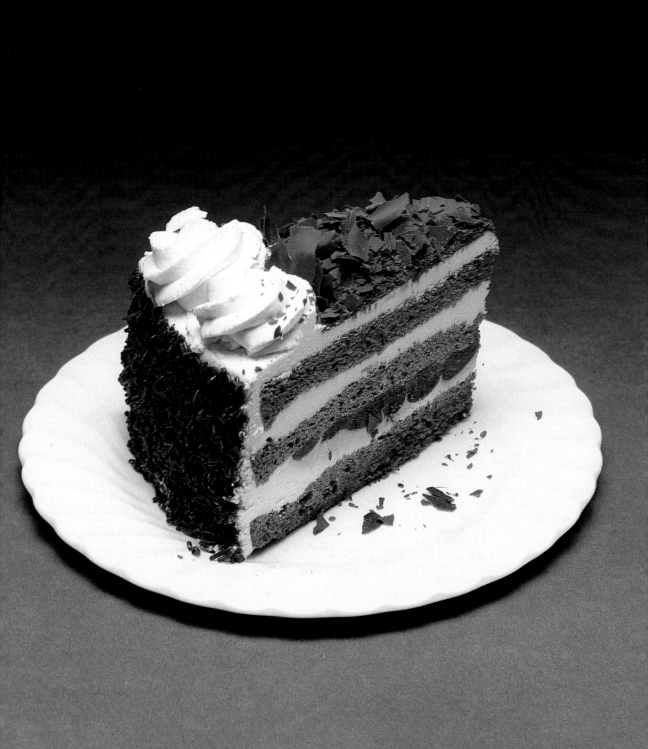

Watching your weight

Energy from food which is not immediately used by the body is stored away as fat. So if you eat more than your daily energy needs, you will gradually put on weight. Regular exercise can help reduce this stored fat, by burning up some of the excess energy stores.

Your actual weight is not too important, as your "healthy" weight will depend on your age, height, sex and general build. (A height and weight chart is shown on page 42.) If you are overweight, it is wise to get rid of this before you develop a real problem.

You can lose weight without starving yourself or starting a fad diet, just by following the recommendations for healthier eating. A good diet, high in fiber, low in sugar and fat, will still fill you up as much as ordinary fattening food, but it will contain far fewer Calories. The fiber is particularly useful as it keeps you feeling full, so you will be less likely to nibble between meals.

Adolescents have special demands on their diet to supply the nutrients needed for healthy growth. If you need to lose a lot of weight, you should consult the doctor before going on a strict diet.

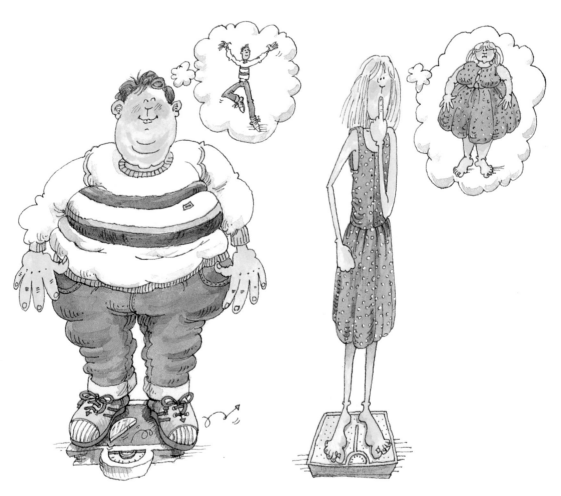

Otherwise, mineral or vitamin deficiency could cause problems.

There is also a risk in adolescence of becoming **anorexic**; that is, having such a fear of becoming overweight that dieting becomes an obsession leading to actual starvation. Some young people develop **bulimia**, a condition in which they eat large amounts of food and then force themselves to vomit to avoid getting fat. There will be none of these problems if you eat just enough of the right sorts of foods.

Our feelings about our body weight do not always reflect the truth. Fat people may feel that they look just right, and will not be concerned about their gradual increase in weight until there is a real health risk. Some people become anorexic, believing that they are grotesquely fat. They then starve themselves, even when it is obvious to others that they are really extremely thin.

Height and weight chart

Boys and girls grow at different rates from childhood to the late teens. At first there are few differences, but boys tend to be taller and heavier than girls by the time they reach their late teens.

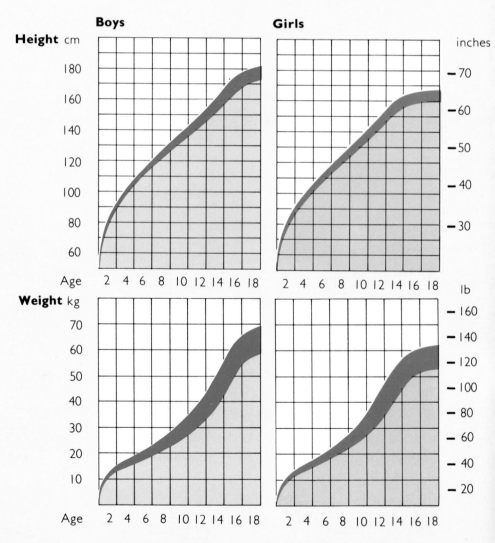

Boys **Girls**

Height cm   inches

Age 2 4 6 8 10 12 14 16 18   2 4 6 8 10 12 14 16 18

Weight kg   lb

Age 2 4 6 8 10 12 14 16 18   2 4 6 8 10 12 14 16 18

A table of foods

This list shows the amounts of fat, sugar, fiber and salt in many common foods. The symbols tell you whether levels are high, medium or low:

● high
◑ medium
○ low

Try to reduce the levels of sugar, fat and salt in your diet, but increase the amount of fiber. The list also gives the energy level of each food in the form of Calories. All the quantities are for 100 g ($3\frac{1}{2}$ oz) of food.

	Energy	Sugar	Fat	Fiber	Salt
Bread					
Wholewheat	216	○	○	●	◑
Brown	233	○	○	◑	◑
White	233	○	○	○	◑
Rice	361	○	○	○	○
Spaghetti	378	○	○	○	○
Breakfast cereals					
Bran flakes	273	◑	○	●	●
Cornflakes	368	○	○	●	●
Muesli	368	●	○	●	○
Cookies and cakes					
Chocolate coated	524	●	●	○	◑
Crackers	440	—	◑	○	◑
Rye crisp	321	○	○	●	○
Doughnuts	349	●	◑	—	○
Fruitcake	332	●	◑	○	○
Shortbread	504	●	●	○	◑

	Energy	Sugar	Fat	Fiber	Salt
Desserts					
Cheesecake	421	◐	●	○	○
Apple crumble	208	●	○	○	○
Ice cream	691	●	○	—	○
Milk and butter					
Full fat milk	76	○	◐	—	○
Skimmed milk	33	○	○	—	○
Butter, salted	740	—	●	—	●
Cream, heavy	447	○	●	—	○
Yogurt					
Natural	52	○	○	—	○
Flavored	81	◐	○	—	○
Cheese					
Cheddar type	406	—	●	—	●
Cottage	96	—	○	—	◐
Processed cheese	311	—	●	—	●
Eggs					
Boiled	147	—	○	—	○
Fats and oils					
Low fat spread	366	—	●	—	◐
Margarine	730	—	●	—	◐
Vegetable oil	899	—	●	—	—
Meat					
Bacon, slice	428	—	●	—	●
Beef, lean	123	—	○	—	○
Hamburger	265	—	●	○	◐
Lamb, leg of	240	—	◐	—	○
Liver	153	—	○	—	○
Pork, leg of	269	—	●	—	○
Pork sausage	367	—	●	○	●
Veal cutlet	215	—	○	—	○
Poultry					
Chicken (meat and skin)	230	—	◐	—	○
Duck (meat, fat and skin)	430	—	●	—	○
Turkey (meat and skin)	145	—	◐	—	○
Fish					
Cod, broiled	95	—	○	—	○
Herring	234	—	◐	—	○
Trout	135	—	○	—	○
Shrimp	107	—	○	—	●
Sauces and pickles					
French dressing	658	○	●	—	●
Mayonnaise	718	○	●	—	◐
Ketchup	98	●	—	—	●

	Energy	Sugar	Fat	Fiber	Salt
Vegetables					
Beans, French	7	○	—	○	○
Broccoli	23	○	—	◐	○
Beans, baked	64	○	●	●	◐
Brussel sprouts	26	○	—	◐	○
Cabbage	26	○	—	◐	○
Cucumber	10	○	○	○	○
Lentils	304	○	○	●	○
Lettuce	12	○	○	○	○
Onions	23	○	—	○	○
Peas, frozen	53	○	○	●	○
Peas, canned	47	○	○	●	◐
Potatoes, boiled	87	○	○	○	○
Potato chips	533	○	●	●	●
Corn, on cob	127	○	○	◐	○
Corn, canned	76	○	○	◐	◐
Tomatoes	14	○	—	○	○
Fruit					
Apples	46	○	—	○	○
Apricots	28	○	—	○	—
Apricots, dried	182	●	—	●	○
Avocado	223	○	●	○	○
Banana	79	◐	○	◐	○
Dates, dried	248	●	—	●	○
Figs, dried	213	●	—	●	○
Grapes	61	◐	—	○	○
Oranges	35	○	—	○	○
Peaches	37	○	—	○	○
Peaches, canned	87	●	—	○	○
Pineapple	46	○	—	○	○
Pineapple, canned	77	●	—	○	○
Prunes	161	●	—	●	○
Strawberries	26	○	—	○	○
Nuts					
Almonds	565	○	◐	●	○
Coconut, shredded	604	○	◐	●	○
Peanut butter	623	○	◐	●	◐
Drinks					
Coffee (no milk)	—	—	—	—	—
Tea (no milk)	—	—	—	—	—
Cola	39	●	—	—	○
Orange juice	33	◐	—	—	○
Tomato juice	16	○	—	—	◐
Candy					
Chocolate, milk	529	●	●	—	○
Chocolate, plain	525	●	●	—	○

Glossary

Additives: substances which are put into food to change it in some way. Additives can improve flavor or color and may also prevent deterioration. They can also be used to make poor quality food look and taste better.

Amino acids: substances produced from our food during digestion. Amino acids are used to make proteins in the body.

Anorexia: loss of appetite. Anorexia nervosa is a serious condition usually affecting adolescents, who eat so little food that they may suffer from starvation.

Appendicitis: inflammation of the appendix, a small finger-like outgrowth at the junction of the small intestine and the large bowel.

Arteries: thick-walled blood vessels carrying blood away from the heart.

Arthritis: condition in which the joints become damaged. It can be very painful.

Bowel: the large intestine in which water is removed from the remains of digested food to produce semi-solid feces.

Bulimia: condition in which a person fears putting on weight, but has a craving for food. They eat, then make themselves vomit so the food will not be digested.

Calcium: important mineral which we obtain from food. It is essential for the growth of healthy bones and teeth.

Calories: measure of the amount of energy obtainable from the food we eat.

Cancer: disease in which body cells multiply out of control.

Carbohydrates: food substances consisting of carbon, hydrogen and oxygen. Sugars, starches and fiber are all forms of carbohydrate.

Cells: small living units from which the whole body is constructed.

Colon: see Bowel.

Constipation: condition in which food material in the intestine moves along very slowly. The feces then become hard and are difficult to pass.

Dental decay: damage to teeth now known to be largely caused by frequent consumption of sugary food and drink.

Diabetes: condition in which the body is unable to make proper use of the sugar we take in from food. The sugar then builds up in the blood and can cause severe illness.

Digestion: the process in which substances in our food are broken down by chemicals in the intestines, so they can be easily absorbed into the body.

Diverticulitis: a condition thought to be caused by lack of fiber in the food, in which after prolonged constipation, small pockets are formed along the bowel which become inflamed.

Fat: food substance from animal or plant foods, which is used as an energy source.

Feces: the solid or semi-solid waste remaining after digestion. Much of its bulk consists of the remains of harmless bacteria from the intestines.

Fiber: indigestible material found in foods of plant origin. Although it cannot be digested, fiber is very important in maintaining the health of the bowel and of other parts of the body.

Gallstones: hard stony deposits in the gall bladder, a small bag in the liver. Gallstones are produced when substances found in the blood are not properly processed by the liver.

Heart disease: any type of illness affecting the heart.

Hemorrhoids: painful swellings in the blood vessels around the anus and rectum which may be caused by a low-fiber diet.

Iron: mineral substance needed for production of healthy red blood cells.

Legumes: dried peas and beans, very rich in fiber and protein.

Minerals: materials found in food which take part in all the chemical processes of the body. Minerals such as calcium, magnesium and phosphorus are important in building bones and teeth.

Nutrients: substances released from food by the process of digestion which can be used by the body for its life processes.

Obesity: overweight, to the point where it can damage health.

Polyunsaturated fat: fat derived mostly from foods of plant origin, which is thought to be less harmful to the heart and arteries than saturated fat.

Protein: food substance found in meat, fish, eggs and dairy products, as well as in some vegetables, nuts and cereals. Foods containing protein are broken down into amino acids during digestion.

Saturated fat: fat found mainly in meat and dairy products which is associated with gradual "furring up" of the arteries if eaten in large amounts.

Sodium: mineral present in large amounts in the blood. It is mainly obtained from common salt.

Sodium chloride: common salt.

Starch: a carbohydrate food material present in plant foods. It is broken down into sugars during digestion.

Stroke: condition in which an artery in the brain bleeds or becomes blocked, causing damage to part of the brain.

Sugar: sweet-tasting carbohydrate nutrient present in many foods.

Urine: liquid waste extracted from the blood by the kidneys. It is stored in the bladder before release.

Vegetarianism: a diet which does not include meat. Some vegetarians also avoid animal products like eggs and butter.

Vitamin: substance obtained from food which helps the chemical processes of the body. Some vitamins are only required in very tiny amounts.

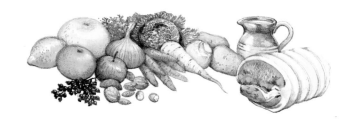

Index